AuthorHouse™
1663 Liberty Drive
Bloomington, IN 47403
www.authorhouse.com
Phone: 1-800-839-8640

First published by AuthorHouse 1/13/2010

ISBN: 978-1-4490-4388-9 (sc)

Printed in the United States of America
Bloomington, Indiana

This book is printed on acid-free paper.

authorHOUSE®

Fighting
Diet Demons

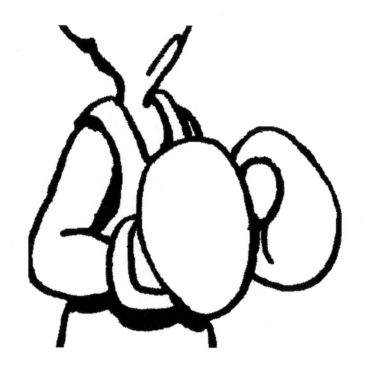

Self Portrait

A look at yourself.

By Sue A. Davis

This book and any programs noted are in no way a replacement for medical advice. The information is for information only and not to be used in place of medical directives The Diet Demon series is to be used for spiritual and scriptural help and not for medical purposes.

I am not a doctor or medical professional and in no way represent myself to be an expert on dieting. This plan is just a fun way to approach getting yourself in a better place with the demons of dieting.

I approach dieting and weight loss with this scripture the main focus of my plan. It does not matter how much you lose, it matters that you are healthy and happy with the temple God has provided for you.

Psalms 139:14-16

14   *I will praise You, for I am fearfully and wonderfully made;*
Marvellous are your works,
And that my soul knows very well.

15   *My frame was not hidden from You,*
When I was made in secret,
And skilfully wrought in the lowest parts of the earth.

16   *Your eyes saw my substance, being yet unformed,*
And in Your book they all were written.
The days fashioned for me,

Spirit Filled Life Bible for Women

Acknowledgement

I want to give thanks to my husband who has encouraged me to finish this series of books. He has been by my side for every pound I have toiled and sweated off. He encouraged me when I was discouraged, comforted me when I cried, held me when I messed up and told me it would be okay and he always reminded me that there is a greater power in my life and all I had to do was to give it to God and he would deal with it. God can take a bad situation and turn it into good, fix what is broken and love us through it all.

This has been a difficult book to finish as I have changed the format several times before I finally came up with an easy to read, easy to understand and helpful way to take a look at our body, mind and spirit. This book can be a fun way to breeze through a weight loss program or just a fun way of sharing accomplishments and discovering what our failures are, and where they come from.

"We *are* fearfully and wonderfully made." It does not matter what we look like, God loves us just the way we are.

Introduction

This workbook is intended for you to get a picture in your head of how you look at yourself. As we proceed through the process your self image will/can change. You will feel better, you will act and react differently. The old feeling of "I still look fat even though I lost 50 pounds", has got to change if you want to feel better about your appearance. You CAN like the way you look. You just need to change your attitude about how you look at yourself.

Start out with the very basics and work from there. Reevaluate yourself every week or so to see if you have made any changes in how you look, act, and react to your lifestyle changes.

Use this tool as a fun way to discover and find yourself. You will also be able to find the comfort level of the skin you are in. God loves us no matter what. So why can't you love what you look like, no matter what.

Work on one exercise a week and by the sixth week you should be able see and feel a big difference.

Have fun and enjoy yourself, this should not be all time consuming and difficult. Look at it as a new adventure.

FIRST

Who am I.

Give a short description of how you look at yourself and who you are.

What do I look like as others see me.

Give a short description of how you think **OTHERS** see you physically.

Why do I want to lose weight.

Give your reasons for wanting to lose weight.

How do I plan on losing weight this time.

Describe how you plan on approaching a weight loss program.

Am I going to be committed?

WHY this time?

NOTES

SECOND

Describe yourself as **YOU** see yourself.

NOTES

Draw a picture of how **YOU** think you look.

This does not have to be perfect, just an idea of how **YOU** see yourself.

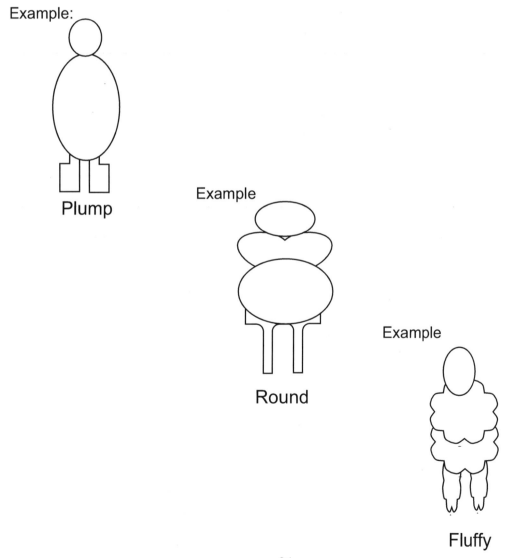

Example:

Plump

Example

Round

Example

Fluffy

Draw a picture of yourself as **YOU** see yourself.

Now draw a picture of how you think **OTHER** people see you.

NOTES

VITAL STATISTICS

Personal Data

Date _____

Name _____

Age _____

Sex _____

Height _____

Weight _____

Goal Weight--Desired _____ Realistic _____

Marital Status _____

Blood Pressure (if known) _____

What type of work do you do. (physical, sedentary etc)

_____

Do you have any handicaps _____

What type of activities do you like to do?

_____

MEN Starting measurements

It is important to measure yourself at the very beginning so you can see the progress.

Have someone measure each location marked.   Hold the tape taught but not too tight.

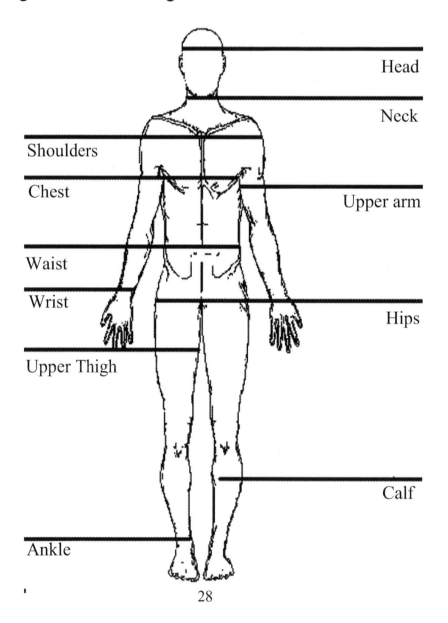

Head

Neck

Shoulders

Chest

Upper arm

Waist

Wrist

Hips

Upper Thigh

Calf

Ankle

WOMEN Starting Measurements.

It is important to measure yourself at the very beginning so you can see the progress.

Have someone measure each location marked.   Hold the

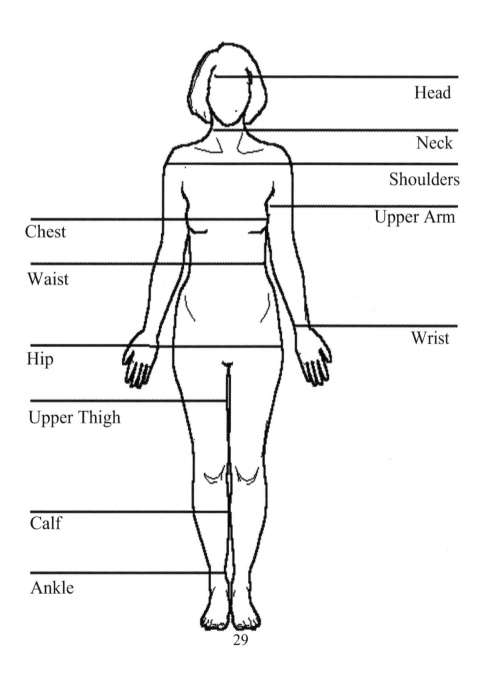

Head

Neck

Shoulders

Upper Arm

Chest

Waist

Wrist

Hip

Upper Thigh

Calf

Ankle

NOTES

Exercise 1

PLANNING

Plan your days.   Start by planning ONE day.   Then graduate to 2 days, 3 days, 4 days, etc. until you can plan for a week at a time.

Plan your meals. Plan the time you will be eating those meals. (This can be a challenge with a family but it is possible). There is absolutely nothing wrong with getting the rest of the family healthy with you.

Start on Sunday. Plan for Monday. Plan your breakfast, lunch, and dinner. Even plan your snacks. It takes very little time to plan meals. The hardest part is to take the time to do it.   Make it a habit. It does get easier, and planning actually works and helps keep you on track.

EXAMPLE

MONDAY
Breakfast 7-8:00 a.m.
    Oatmeal, Fruit, coffee, toast.
Snack 10:00 a.m.
    Apple
Lunch 11:30-12:30
    Vegetables, protein, Carbohydrate, coffee/tea/water/diet soda.
Snack 2:00 p.m.
    Raw veggies or fruit
Dinner 5:00 p.m.
    Vegetables, protein, (carbohydrate if not at lunch), salad.
Snack 7-8:00 p.m.
    Fruit or raw veggies (I like frozen berries)

This is just a sample day, the food plan all depends on which program you are following. This sample was taken from the Diet Demons Plan. Try to eat at the same time every day and you will find it easier to follow any plan.

MONDAY

Breakfast TIME

Food choices

Snack TIME

Food choices

Lunch TIME

Food choices

Snack TIME

Food choices

Dinner TIME

Food choices

Snack TIME

Food choices

TUESDAY

Breakfast TIME

Food choices

Snack TIME

Food choices

Lunch TIME

Food choices

Snack TIME

Food choices

Dinner TIME

Food choices

Snack TIME

Food choices

WEDNESDAY

Breakfast TIME

Food choices

Snack TIME

Foods choices

Lunch TIME

Food choices

Snack TIME

Food choices

Dinner TIME

Food choices

Snack TIME

Food choices

THURSDAY

Breakfast TIME

Food choices

Snack TIME

Foods choices

Lunch TIME

Food choices

Snack TIME

Food choices

Dinner TIME

Food choices

Snack TIME

Food choices

FRIDAY

Breakfast TIME

Food choices

Snack TIME

Foods choices

Lunch TIME

Food choices

Snack TIME

Food choices

Dinner TIME

Food choices

Snack TIME

Food choices

SATURDAY

Breakfast TIME

Food choices

Snack TIME

Foods choices

Lunch TIME

Food choices

Snack TIME

Food choices

Dinner TIME

Food choices

Snack TIME

Food choices

SUNDAY

Breakfast TIME ....

Food choices ....

Snack TIME ....

Foods choices ....

Lunch TIME ....

Food choices ....

Snack TIME ....

Food choices ....

Dinner TIME ....

Food choices ....

Snack TIME ....

Food choices ....

REMEMBER: Take the time to sit down and plan your week. If you plan ahead there will be no surprises.   Yes! You can even eat out at a restaurant if you plan ahead for this.   Please see the Fighting Diet Demons Book for information on eating out.

MEN

It is important to measure yourself at the very beginning so you can see the progress.

Have someone measure each location marked. Hold the tape taught but not too tight.

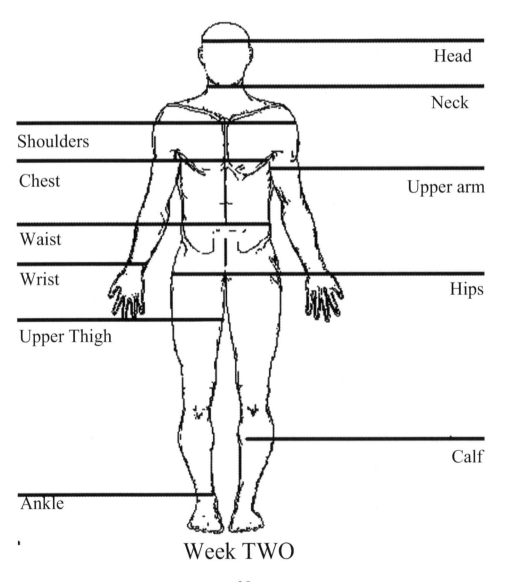

Head

Neck

Shoulders

Chest

Upper arm

Waist

Wrist

Hips

Upper Thigh

Calf

Ankle

Week TWO

WOMEN (same as for men)

It is important to measure yourself at the very beginning so you can see the progress.

Have someone measure each location marked. Hold the tape taught but not too tight.

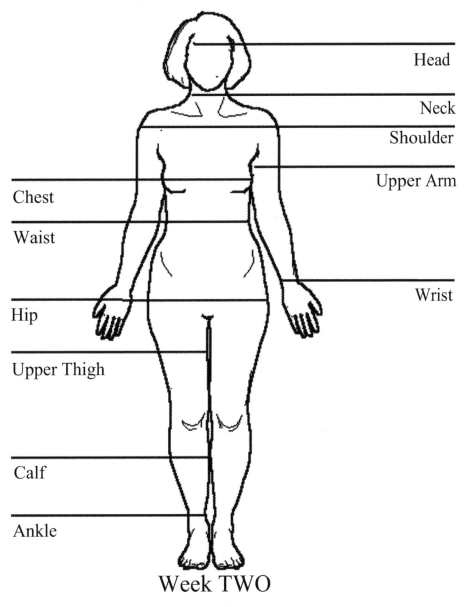

Head

Neck

Shoulder

Upper Arm

Chest

Waist

Wrist

Hip

Upper Thigh

Calf

Ankle

Week TWO

NOTES

Exercise 2

Exercise

Walk up a flight of stairs, or across the room.
Describe how you feel. (How do your legs, calves,
ankles, hips, and back feel?)

Now using a 10 pound bag of potatoes (or anything that weighs 10 pounds), place 10 pounds under each arm and walk up the same flight of stairs or across the room again. Again describe how you feel in your arms, legs, back, and the calves of your legs.

Now for an easy one. Bend over and tie your shoes.
Describe how you do this. Do you turn to the side, or
do you have to put your foot on a chair to reach your
feet?   Describe in detail how you do this.

Cross your legs as you are sitting in a chair. How does this feel. Do you feel or look like you are uncomfortable?

_____

_____

_____

_____

_____

_____

_____

_____

_____

_____

_____

Repeat these exercises weekly. You will be amazed at the difference you will notice as you lose a few extra pounds.

NOTES

MEN

It is important to measure yourself at the very beginning so you can see the progress.

Have someone measure each location marked. Hold the tape taught but not too tight.

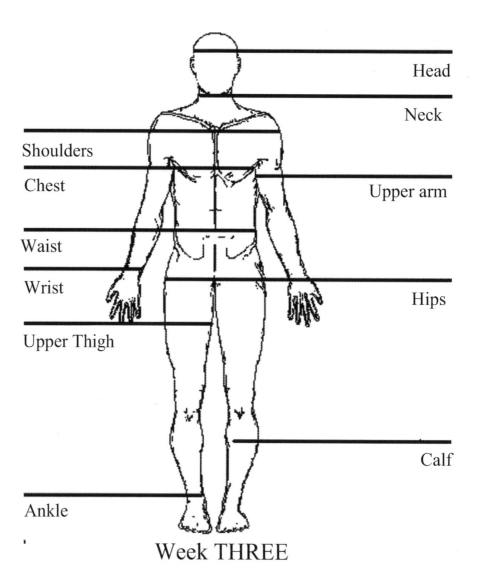

Head

Neck

Shoulders

Chest

Upper arm

Waist

Wrist

Hips

Upper Thigh

Calf

Ankle

Week THREE

WOMEN (same as for men)

It is important to measure yourself at the very beginning so you can see the progress.

Have someone measure each location marked. Hold the tape taught but not too tight.

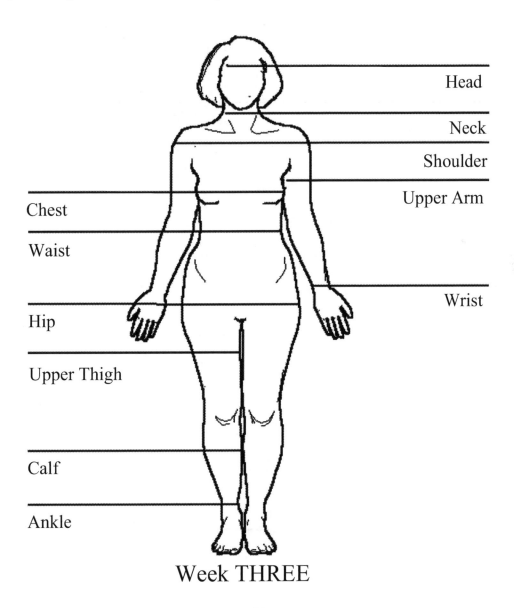

Week THREE

NOTES

Exercise 3

Exercise

Find a scripture or scriptures that you can rely on to help get you through the tough times. Write it down and carry it in your pocket.

If need be, have it printed on a business card, set it out in different places to remind you that you are trimming that temple of God into a stream lined vessel of a healthy child of God. We may be of a cathedral size now but when we reach chapel size we can be much more active and outgoing that we can take on enough chapel size projects to fill that old cathedral image.

My favorite scriptures:

1. I can do all things in he who strengthens me.   Phillipians 4:13
2. I am fearfully and wonderfully made.

1. ....

2. ....

3. ....

MEN

It is important to measure yourself at the very beginning so you can see the progress.

Have someone measure each location marked. Hold the tape taught but not too tight.

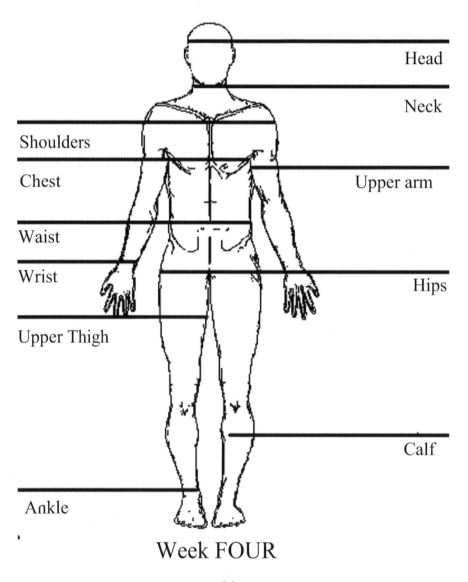

Head

Neck

Shoulders

Chest

Upper arm

Waist

Wrist

Hips

Upper Thigh

Calf

Ankle

Week FOUR

WOMEN (same as for men)

It is important to measure yourself at the very beginning so you can see the progress.

Have someone measure each location marked. Hold the tape taught but not too tight.

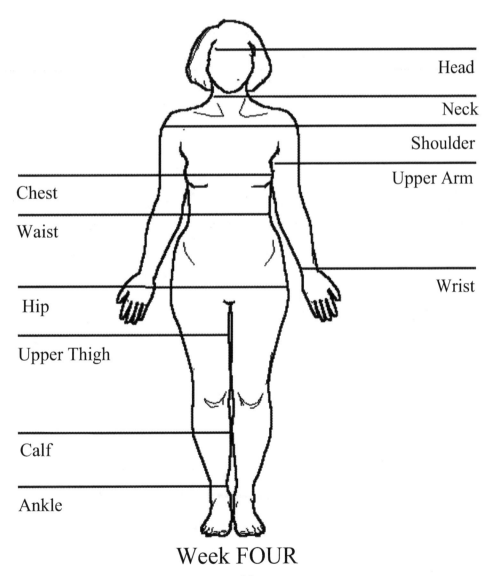

Head
Neck
Shoulder
Upper Arm
Chest
Waist
Wrist
Hip
Upper Thigh
Calf
Ankle

Week FOUR

NOTES

Exercise 4

Exercise

Find a food from the bible that will help with your weight loss. There are a couple of them.   (You will find more information on these in the *Fighting Diet Demons* book). Jesus never ate junk food. Lets take his example and follow in his footsteps for a better healthy lifestyle. He did not eat junk and he did not make junk, so let's not trash the bodies he gave us stewardship over.

LIST the foods Jesus ate and how you think they were intended for our health and well being.

_____

_____

_____

_____

_____

_____

_____

_____

_____

_____

_____

_____

MEN

It is important to measure yourself at the very beginning so you can see the progress.

Have someone measure each location marked. Hold the tape taught but not too tight.

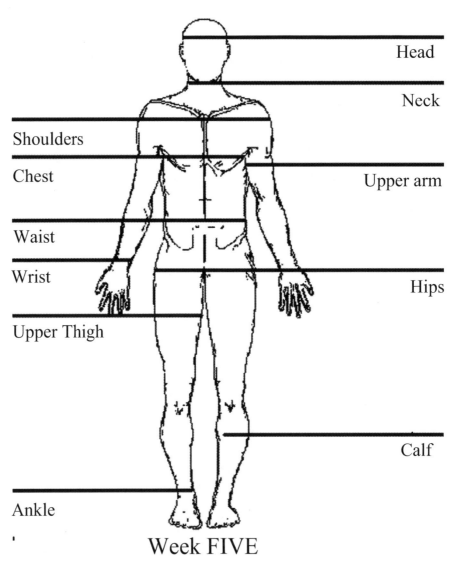

Head

Neck

Shoulders

Chest

Upper arm

Waist

Wrist

Hips

Upper Thigh

Calf

Ankle

Week FIVE

WOMEN (same as for men)

It is important to measure yourself at the very beginning so you can see the progress.

Have someone measure each location marked. Hold the tape taught but not too tight.

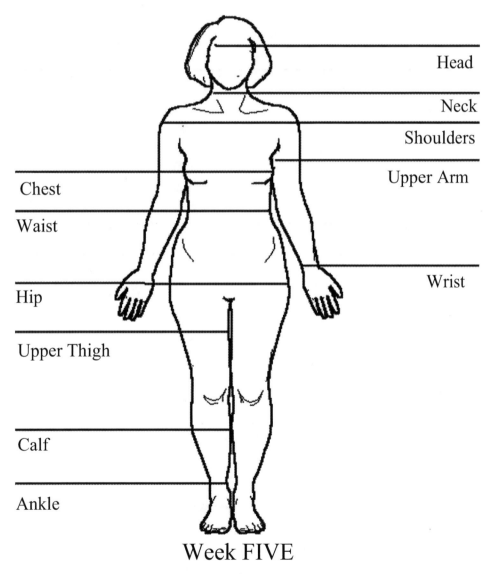

Head

Neck

Shoulders

Upper Arm

Chest

Waist

Wrist

Hip

Upper Thigh

Calf

Ankle

Week FIVE

NOTES

Exercise 5

Exercise

Work on your bondage and addictions.

Get rid of the shackles and chains of bondage that keep you from succeeding in trimming down and living a healthy life.

What are my chains of bondage?

How do I plan on getting rid of them?

NOTES

MEN

It is important to measure yourself at the very beginning so you can see the progress.

Have someone measure each location marked. Hold the tape taught but not too tight.

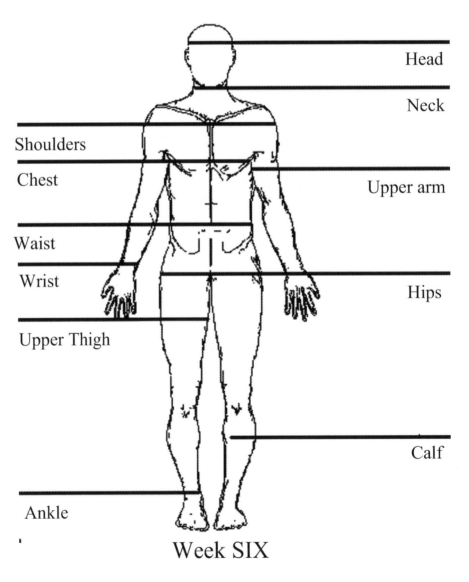

Week SIX

WOMEN (same as for men)

It is important to measure yourself at the very beginning so you can see the progress.

Have someone measure each location marked. Hold the tape taught but not too tight.

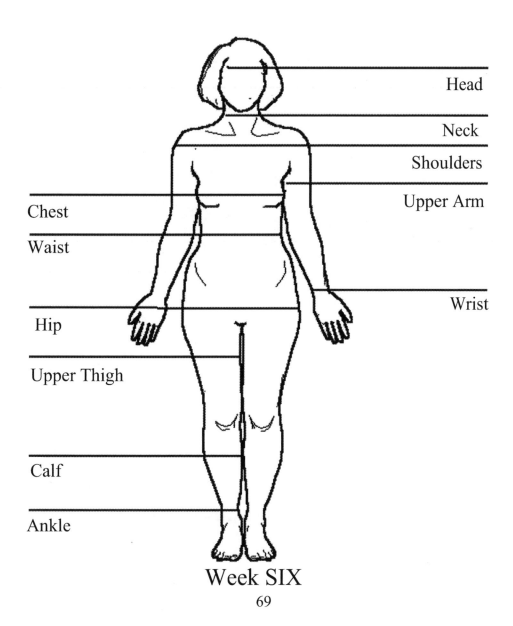

Week SIX

NOTES

Exercise 6

Exercise

Start something new. Make some new habits that include exercise.

•Park a little further away from work and walk.

•Walk to work.

•Walk the mall. (This does not mean STROLLING through the mall).

•While sitting at your desk do leg lifts and waist bends.

•While lying in bed do leg lifts.

•While talking on the phone do side bends.

•Do leg stretches while waiting for some one to answer the phone.

•Do neck stretches and chin lifts while driving.

•Get out of bed, greet the day to waist stretches and toe touches.

•While watching TV do toning exercises.

•You don't have to break a sweat as long as you do something every day.

Have you ever noticed how well toned a cats body is? All they do for conditioning are stretching exercises. (Have you ever seen a cat break out in a sweat from over working itself.)

It is as simple as lifting a can of vegetables (Kind of like dumbbells) every day. Lift them up or pull them up, both functions tone the upper arms. Simple exercises for toning help you feel good as well as help improve your stamina. (You don't have to exercise until you hurt, or are out of breath.) If you need to do armchair exercises then do them.   Just find something in your comfort zone and make it a habit.

Find and list all the exercises you can do that will fit in with your lifestyle.

NOTES

MEN

It is important to measure yourself at the very beginning so you can see the progress.

Have someone measure each location marked. Hold the tape taught but not too tight.

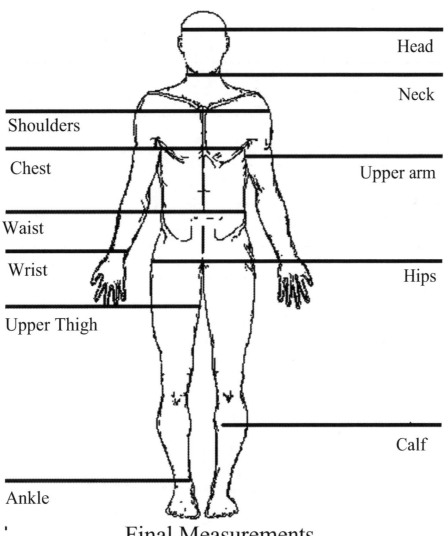

Head

Neck

Shoulders

Chest

Upper arm

Waist

Wrist

Hips

Upper Thigh

Calf

Ankle

Final Measurements

WOMEN (same as for men)

It is important to measure yourself at the very beginning so you can see the progress.

Have someone measure each location marked. Hold the tape taught but not too tight.

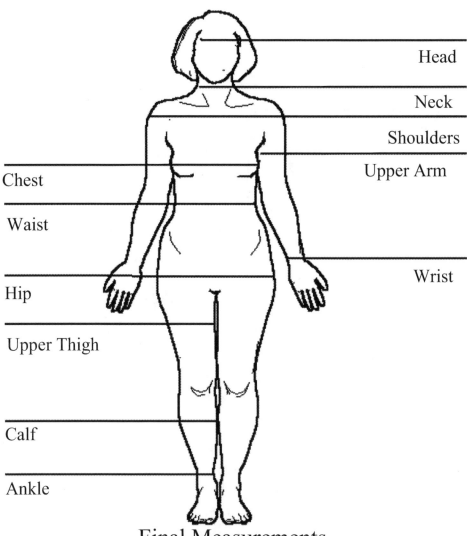

Head

Neck

Shoulders

Upper Arm

Chest

Waist

Wrist

Hip

Upper Thigh

Calf

Ankle

Final Measurements

SUMMARY

Now that you have taken a closer look at some of the ways to conquer the demons that keep you on a path to personal health deterioration, how do you feel?

Did you lose any unwanted pounds?

Were you hungry?

Did you discover something about yourself that you did not know before?

Have you taken a good hard look at how you perceive your appearance and your overall health?

Did you read the book *Fighting Diet Demons*?

Did you utilize the *Fighting Diet Demons Journal.* Using a Journal is yet another tool that is very beneficial to success in any weight control program.

Please use the last few pages to write down your thoughts and progress from these workbook exercises.

Authors comments:

I am currently working on a facilitator instruction workbook if you would like to utilize this Self Portrait Workbook as a Bible study program in your Church.

FINAL TOTALS

Total Weeks Completed _____

	Beginning	Ending	Difference
Weight			
Blood Pressure			
Head			
Neck			
Shoulders			
Chest			
Upper Arm			
Waist			
Wrist			
Hips			
Upper thigh			
Calf			
Ankle			

Be blessed and keep God in your journey to good health.
God loves you... and He loves you
JUST THE WAY YOU ARE.

Always remember ... Psalms 193:14

NOTES

NOTES

NOTES